10-Minute Primer
Chinese Kung Fu (Wushu)

other books in the same series

10-Minute Primer Qigong
Zhou Qingjie
ISBN 978 1 84819 212 6

10-Minute Primer Shaolin Quan
Zhou Qigong
ISBN 978 1 84819 214 0

10-Minute Primer Tai Ji Quan
Zhou Qingjie
ISBN 978 1 84819 215 7

10-Minute Primer

CHINESE KUNG FU (WUSHU)

Zhou Qingjie

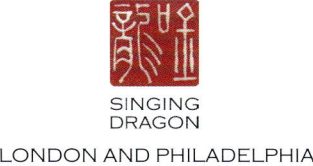

SINGING
DRAGON

LONDON AND PHILADELPHIA

This edition published in 2014
by Singing Dragon
an imprint of Jessica Kingsley Publishers
73 Collier Street
London N1 9BE, UK
and
400 Market Street, Suite 400
Philadelphia, PA 19106, USA

www.singingdragon.com

First published by Foreign Languages Press, Beijing, China, 2009

Library of Congress Cataloging in Publication Data
Zhou, Qingjie.
  10-minute primer Chinese wushu / Zhou Qingjie.
    pages cm
  Originally published: Beijing : Foreign Language Press, 2009.
  ISBN 978-1-84819-213-3 (alk. paper)
  1. Kung fu. I. Title. II. Title: Ten minute primer Chinese wushu.
  GV1114.7.Z5 2014
  796.815'9--dc23
                            2013037074

British Library Cataloguing in Publication Data
A CIP catalogue record for this book is available from the British Library

ISBN 978 1 84819 213 3

Printed and bound in China

PRONUNCIATION GUIDE

中　zhōng—similar to *jung* in *jung*le
国　guó—the sound g plus war
武　wǔ—*woo*
术　shù—*shoe*

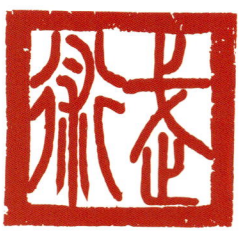

❮CONTENTS❯

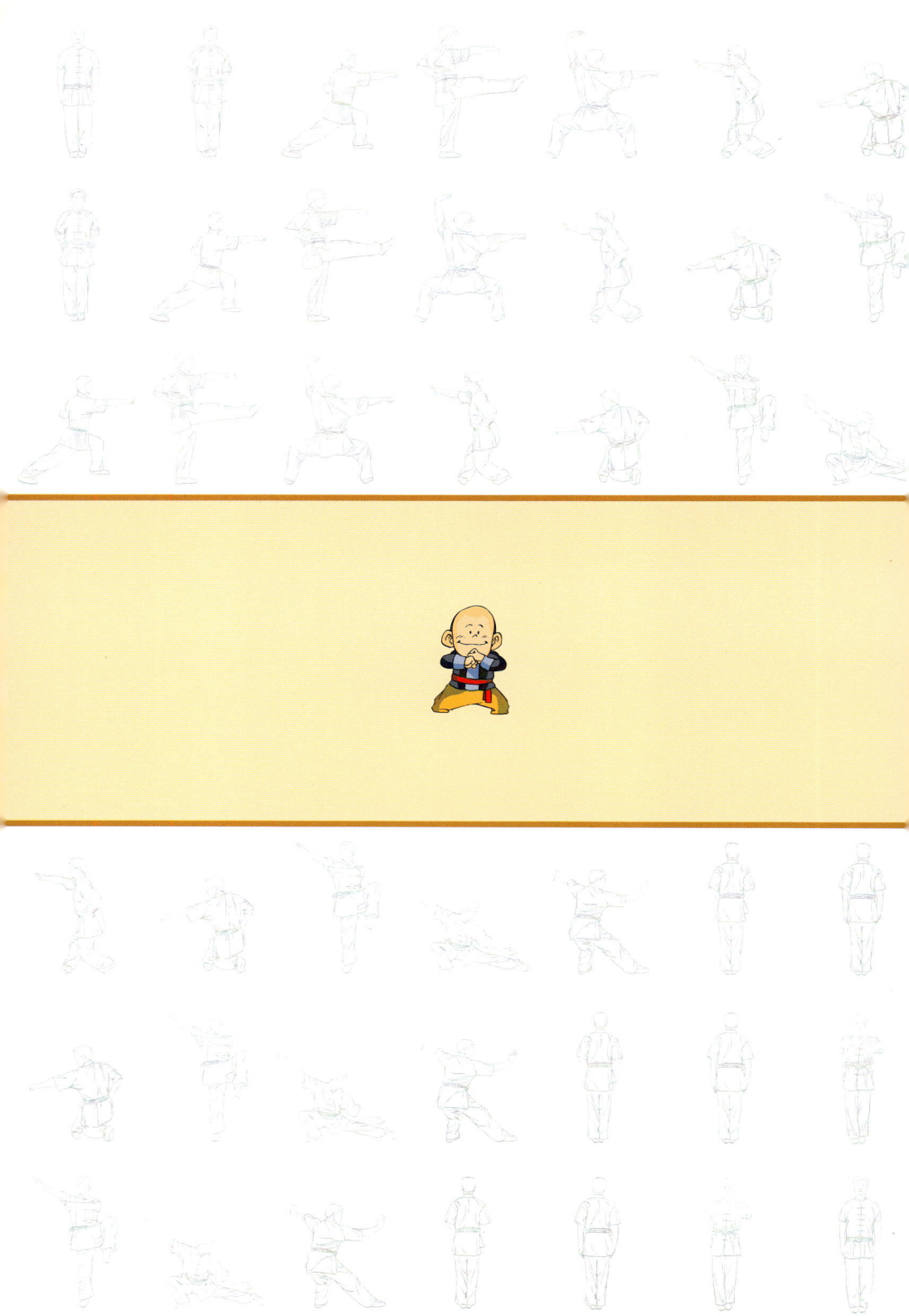

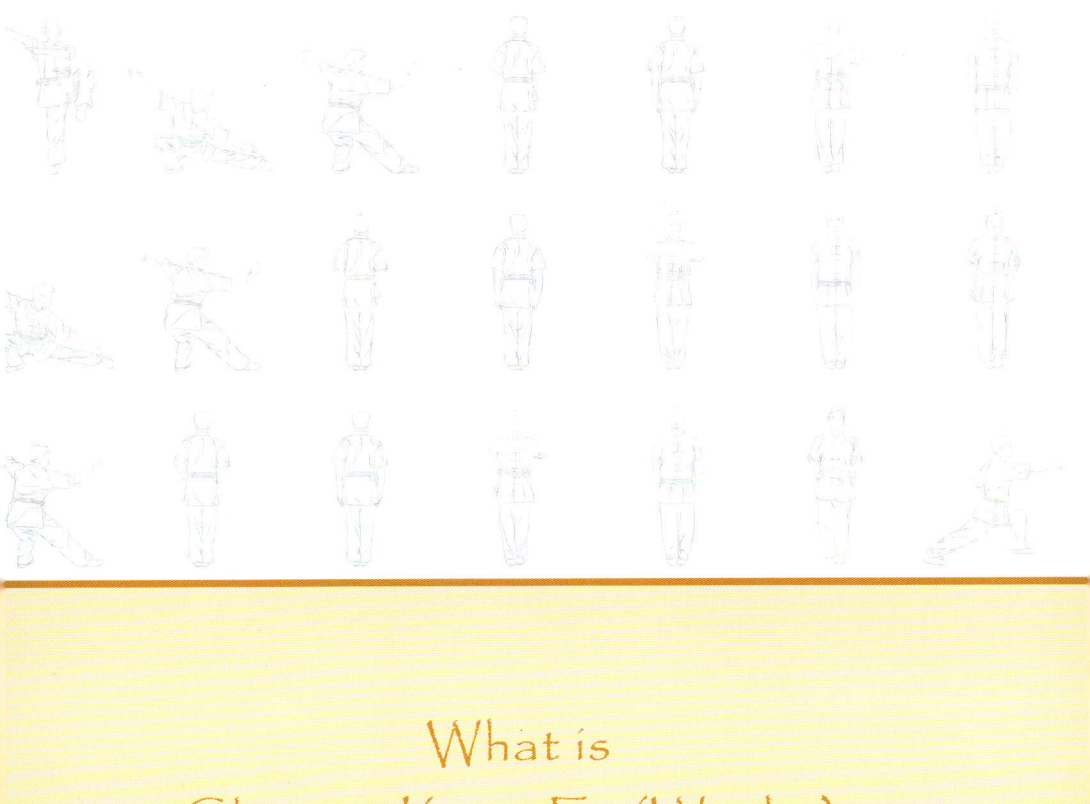

What is
Chinese Kung Fu (Wushu)?

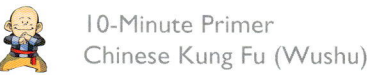
Chinese kung fu or wushu

Chinese kung fu or wushu is a traditional Chinese sport, with the art of attack and defense as its main content and the routines, fighting and practice of skills as the exercise forms, which pays equal attention to internal and external cultivation.

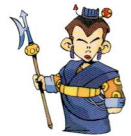

Wu 武

You can see a picture of the Chinese character 戈 ge (dagger-axe) contained in wu, which means "martial." According to the *Origins of Chinese Characters, wu* means "to stop fighting." It means using *wu* to forbid violence, eliminate turmoil, and stop fighting, thus seeking stability and peace.

Wu also has another meaning: "The best of martial strength is demonstrated by compassion and reputation—convince people without the use of arms."

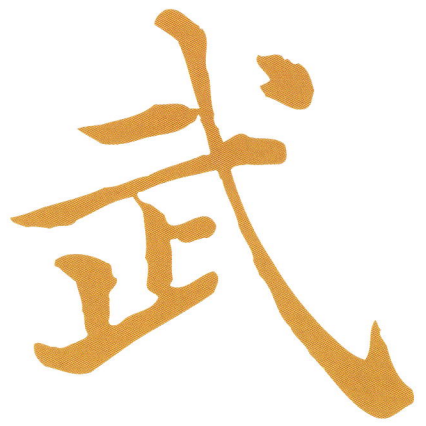

Shu 术

*S*hu refers to art, technique, methods and tactics.

Kung fu

The word "kung fu" originated from "*da gongfu,*" as pronounced in the Guangdong dialect, meaning "practicing wushu." As people from Guangdong early on began to teach wushu in other parts of the world, and since Bruce Lee, the world's kung fu master, often used the word "kung fu" in his martial arts movies, people in many countries and regions became more familiar with "kung fu" than with "wushu." However, "kung fu" and "wushu" are in fact the same thing, with the word "wushu" being formally more standard.

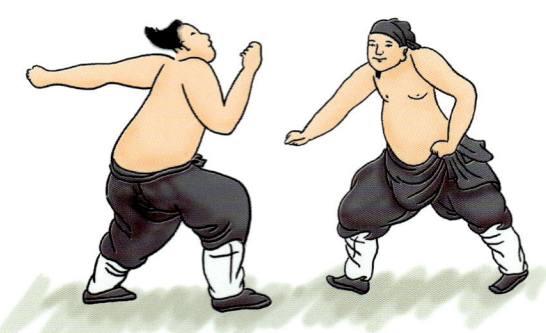

Thirty-two Changquan ("long boxing") technique from
Ming Dynasty General Qi Jiguang's *A Treatise on Efficiency*

"Gongfu," the standard Chinese spelling of kung fu, is also another word for "time." For example, there is a Chinese saying: "If you have gongfu (time), please come." If you want to have a good mastery of gongfu, you must persevere in practicing hard at it on the basis of using correct methodology, acknowledging it is possible to achieve only after years of consistent effort. Today, people often use "practicing wushu" and "practicing gongfu" interchangeably.

"Gongfu is the crystallization of time and sweat."

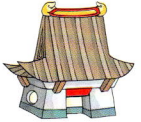

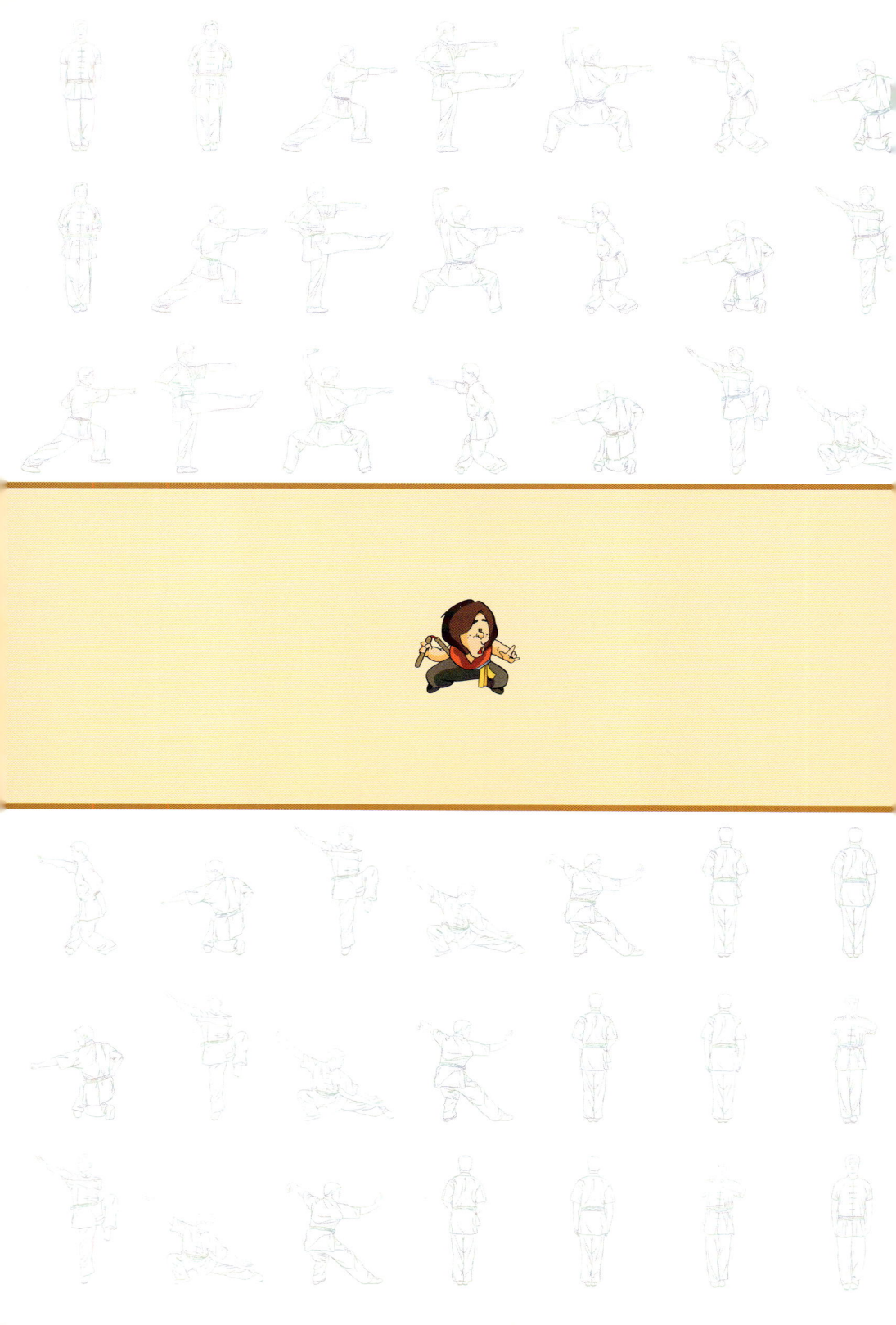

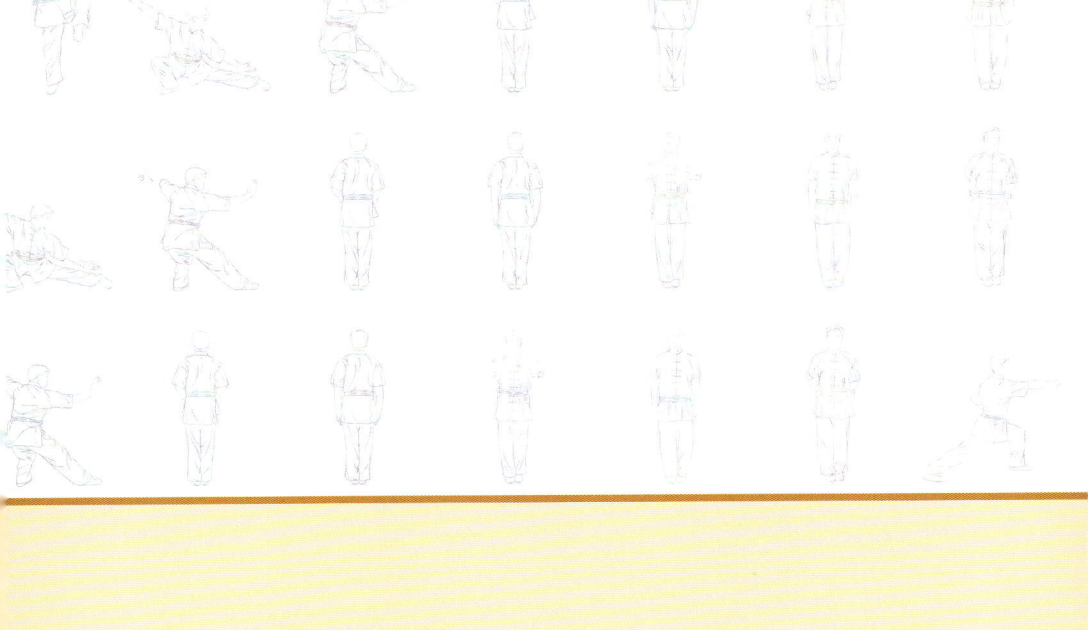

What Else besides Bruce Lee Should You Know?

Chinese kung fu films

Chinese kung fu films have made a major contribution to world film. For decades these movies have been very popular in all parts of the world.

The rapid rise of Chinese kung fu films generally benefited from the martial arts novels that had been very popular for centuries. The Shanghai Star Co. Ltd. produced the first Chinese kung fu film, *Set the Honglian Temple on Fire* in 1928. But no further kung fu films were produced in mainland China in the subsequent period because of war and political turmoil. However, the 1940s and 1950s saw the first upsurge of kung fu film production in Hong Kong. For example, there were as many as 77 films in the Huang Feihong series. Chinese kung fu films were born on the mainland, but flourished in Hong Kong.

The development of Chinese kung fu films reached its zenith in the period from the 1960s to the 1990s. This period was not only an important stage of the internationalization of Chinese kung fu films, but also saw the emergence of many important directors of martial arts films (e.g. Hu Jinquan, Zhang Che and Liu Jialiang) and international stars (e.g. Bruce Lee, Jackie Chan and Jet Li).

Among Chinese kung fu film stars up to the present, the most influential and enduring was none other than Bruce Lee. The unyielding and dauntless spirit of fearing no brutal enemy and preferring death over submission, along with the Chinese martial arts that Bruce Lee demonstrated in every one of his kung fu films, have left an indelible impression on every cinemagoer in the world. In fact, the core value of the Chinese kung fu films represented by Bruce Lee is upholding justice and persisting in efforts to pursue the true, the good and the beautiful.

It needs to be especially noted that the word "kung fu" was included in English dictionaries entirely because of Bruce Lee's global influence. It is incredible that in the decades after Bruce Lee became popular and even after his death, his fans in many countries still cherish the memory of their favorite hero—Bruce Lee. Bruce Lee seems to have become the embodiment of and synonym for "kung fu."

The 21st century has ushered in a new period of Chinese kung fu films. Several Chinese martial arts films have made a major impact on world film. These include *Crouching Tiger, Hidden Dragon*, *Hero*, and *Seven Swords*. Yuan Heping and Yuan Kui, two world-class wushu instructors, successfully created a space for the development of Chinese kung fu films in popular culture. Hollywood's *Matrix*, *Kill Bill* and *Dead or Alive* are some of their most famous masterpieces.

The film *Crouching Tiger, Hidden Dragon*, winner of the Oscar for Best Picture demonstrates chivalrous swordsmen and swordswomen fighting atop bamboo trees, sometimes resembling lightening and thunder, and other times more like the delicate bamboo leaves. These gongfu feats, which had earlier only been seen in Chinese gongfu novels, captivated moviegoers around the world. Above all, such memorable scenes provided artistic thrills full of Eastern philosophical flavor to Western cinemagoers, who were more used to military confrontations between two armies. Who would have thought that blood-filled fight scenes could also be so artistically beautiful and entertaining!

Wushu in traditional Chinese operas

Traditional Chinese opera uses "singing, acting, speaking and fighting" to create a unique artistic performance. Whether in form or in content, the "fighting" aspect is closely related to movements of attack and defense in wushu. Moreover, the "eighteen kinds of weapons" used in wushu have been used on the theatrical stage to display the fighting and battle scenes as required by the plot. After years of constant development and refinement, Peking opera performers include *wusheng* (actor playing a martial role), *wudan* (actress playing a martial role), *wujing* (painted-face actor playing a martial role), and *wuchou* (acrobatic clown).

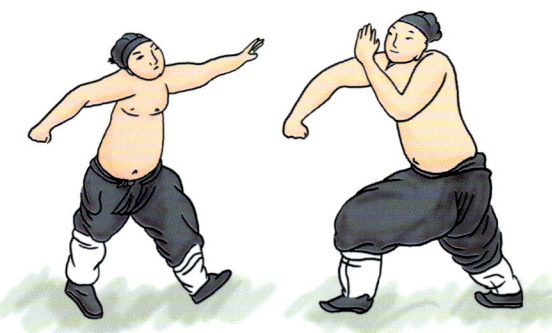

Thirty-two Changquan ("long boxing") technique from
Ming Dynasty General Qi Jiguang's *A Treatise on Efficiency*

Many opera masters have mastered effective wushu skills, with some even reaching the highest attainments in wushu. For example, Tan Xinpei, reputed as the "king of performers" in Peking opera for his superb skill that assimilated the special techniques of all schools, was originally an armed escort. When he acted as Shi Xiu (hero from *Outlaws of the Marsh*) in the opera *Mount Cuiping*, he performed Liuhe swordplay using a real sword, with astonishingly superb skill that often inspired deafening cheering from theater-going crowds. Gai Jiaotian, a famous *wusheng* actor, was not only

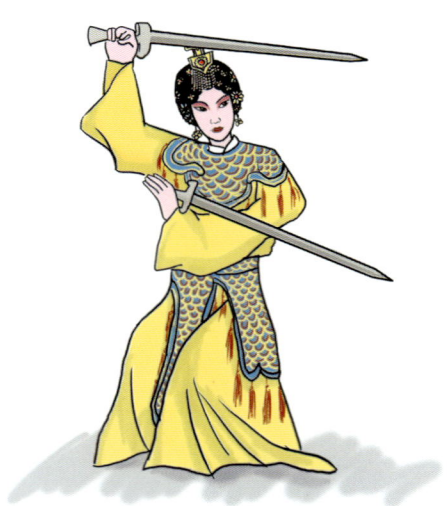

Farewell My Concubine

a spellbinding performer of acrobatic fighting on the stage, but also a wushu master. He not only knew how to perform with weapons as well as barehanded fighting, but could also turn the best wushu into a skillful stage art, to form a unique school of theatrical fighting of his own. The swordsmanship display performed by Mei Lanfang, the world-renowned Peking opera master, in *Farewell My Concubine*, was a good fusion of the charms of the movements of Xingyi (form and will) quan (a form of gongfu), which is based on the fighting movements of 12 animals, and Taiji swordplay in wushu. Cheng Yanqiu, whose name has gone down in Chinese performing-arts history, successfully blended wushu techniques into theatrical acting, and created unique dance steps in his graceful water-sleeve dance, passing on a valuable artistic heritage to later generations. There are far too many examples for it to be possible to cite them all in this book.

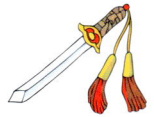

Religious wushu culture

Whether in Chinese Buddhism or Daoism, or the secret religions that existed among people through Chinese history, all are closely related with wushu. Shaolin wushu and Wudang wushu are, however, the most influential among Chinese religious wushu schools.

Shaolin Temple wushu culture

Shaolin Temple is the ancestral temple of the Chan (or Zen) Sect of Chinese Buddhism. It is located on Mount Songshan in Dengfeng County, Henan Province.

The Shaolin Temple gradually developed its own extensive cultural system with distinctive features. The system embraces Chan (sitting in meditation), wushu, medicine, ancient architecture, historical literature and books, as well as food and drink, and daily life. The most salient features of Shaolin culture are: integration of Chan meditation and wushu, with wushu as the embodiment of Chan; medicine as supporting wings of wushu; and the collection of the best from all other schools. There are two prevalent beliefs regarding the origins of Shaolin gongfu: one, it was created by Dharma; and two, it was created by Huiguang and Zeng Chou, disciples of Batuo, the founder of the Shaolin Temple.

According to the literature published by the Shaolin Temple, the illustrative chart of Shaolin quan, handed down in the temple, records 708 routines of Shaolin quan, and 156 sets of exercises (e.g. "72 Unique Skills," *qin na* or the skill of incapacitating an opponent by manipulating his joints and acupoints, bone disjointing, *qigong*). In the Chinese world, the most familiar Shaolin gongfu includes Yi Jin Jing (Tendon-Muscle Strengthening Exercises), Tie Bu Shan (Iron Cloth Shirt [that no weapon can harm]), Shaolin cudgel, and Shaolin bone dislocation.

Today, Shaolin wushu has spread all over world, with disciples found everywhere. Wushu lovers even include an English royal family member, the French premier, the

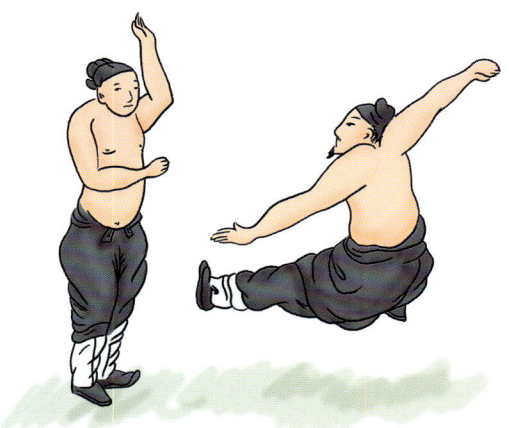

Thirty-two Changquan ("long boxing") technique from
Ming Dynasty General Qi Jiguang's *A Treatise on Efficiency*

Russian president, a Japanese cabinet member, and a US congressman. Since 1987, the Temple has sent groups of martial arts monks to more than 60 countries. Today, it has set up six academies in other countries, and more than 50 countries and regions have established Shaolin schools and groups. Shaolin gongfu has become a unique social and cultural phenomenon, and has played an important role in cultural exchanges between China and other countries, unparalleled by other sports.

Publication: *Chan Lu*.

Major sporting event: International Shaolin Wushu Festival.

Mount Wudang wushu culture

Mount Wudang is considered one of the sacred birthplaces of Chinese Daoism, also being the cradle of legendary Wudang quan—a kind of *neijia* gongfu that pays more attention to the inner work and strength. It is also famous for its incomparable scenery, and described as the No. 1 "Mountain of Immortals" in the world.

Since ancient times, Daoism has advocated practicing the Dao (Way) with indifference to fame and fortune, with restraint in behavior, and boxing to be practiced only by its disciples. This was a major obstacle to any widespread promotion of Wudang gongfu. Moreover, Daoist wushu was also limited by its religious discipline of "speaking of the founder rather than the masters." This has made it difficult for others to study it in any depth.

Wudang quan derived its name from Wudang Mountain. It is one of the major schools of Chinese martial arts. In the wushu world, there is a saying: "Shaolin is respected in the north and Wudang in the south." Its characteristics include: checking motion with stillness, overcoming the strong with the soft, subduing the long with the short, stopping the swift with the slow, directing the *qi* (energy) with the will, and

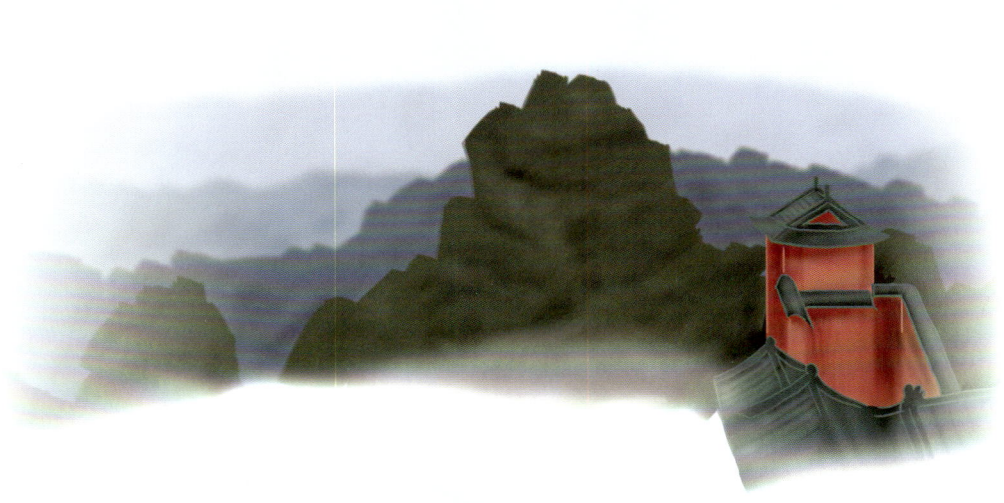

motivating the body with *qi*. Wudang school martial arts include Taiji quan and Wuji quan; and Wudang weapons include Wudang swordplay, Baihong swordplay and Liuhe (six-conformity) spear play.

Publication: *Wudang*.

Major sporting event: Chinese Wudang Cultural and Wushu Festival, and International Wudang Quan Exchange Fair.

Chinese wushu culture regards Shaolin as exemplary of *waijia* or external gongfu (stress on muscles, bone and skin), and Wudang as representative of *neijia* or internal gongfu (stress on spirit, energy and mind). Wudang wushu culture is not as widespread as Shaolin wushu culture, but its profound and complex Daoist way of maintaining good health gives it added mysterious appeal. It should be particularly noted that both Shaolin gongfu and Wudang wushu are included in the First List of Intangible Cultural Heritage under State Protection, published by the State Council of China in May 2006.

Chivalrous culture

Chivalrous swordsmen

China had a profound reclusive culture in ancient times. Great figures who had attained a deep understanding of worldly affairs often later chose to live alone as hermits and be independent, rather than to swim and sink in everyday affairs. As Chen Wangting, the founder of Chen-style Taiji quan, advised: "Practice Taiji quan in leisure time, and do farm work in the busy season." It is clear that the genuine chivalrous swordsmen and wushu

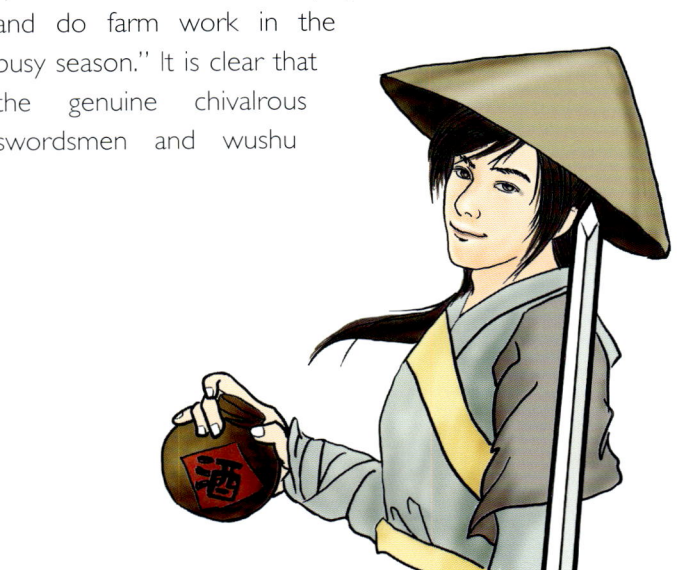

masters usually concealed themselves in obscure places, and gongfu was simply a tool they used to meet the needs of their cultural life.

The personal values of gongfu masters were: value justice and help others at the risk of their own lives, cherish brotherhood and personal loyalty, and never break a promise...

"The most important thing for a chivalrous swordsman is to serve the nation and the people." The great integrity of chivalrous swordsmen was what the ordinary people did not have and aspired to. However, the path to the spiritual realm of the chivalrous swordsmen was gongfu.

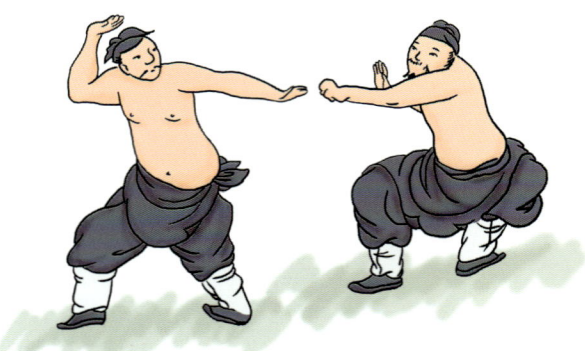

Thirty-two Changquan ("long boxing") technique from Ming Dynasty General Qi Jiguang's *A Treatise on Efficiency*

Novels of chivalry

China had heroic novels from ancient times. Among the best-known novels are: *Outlaws of the Marsh*, *Tales of Chivalrous Swordsmen*, and *Stories of Young Heroes and Heroines*. *Outlaws of the Marsh* became an eternal Chinese classic. In modern times, 600 to 700 published novels of chivalry have been recorded. The contemporary novels written by Jin Yong, Liang Yusheng and Gu Long are very popular in the Chinese world.

The value of the heroic novels lies in the fact that it is a fictitious world carefully woven by the authors, who have made use of the extraordinary military skills of gallant chivalrous swordsmen and swordswomen to depict the power of idealism. It often has larger-than-life significance. The root cause of the Chinese chivalrous complex is the longing for realization of personal worth in life, along with resistance from the innermost heart to social injustice. Novels of chivalry can be regarded as "fairytales for adults."

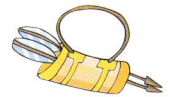

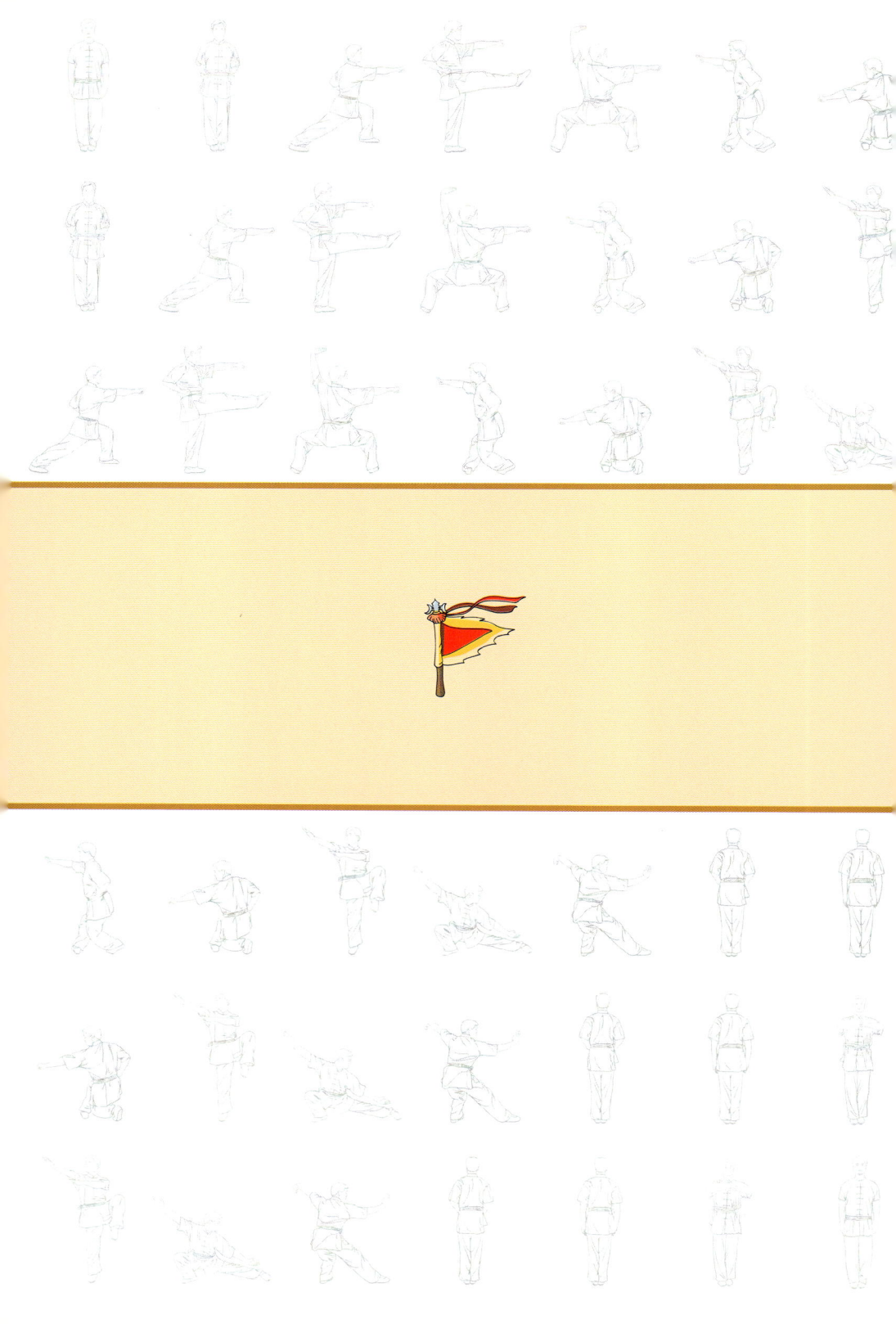

Wushu: From Stone-Age Battles to Modern Fantasies

China's earliest "hidden weapon"— rope trap to trip beasts

In remote times, people used a hunting device called "rope to trip beasts." It was a long rope with one end tied to a stone ball. The hunter, with the other end tied around his arm, would chase a wild animal and cast the stone ball towards the animal as he approached it. The stone would pull at the

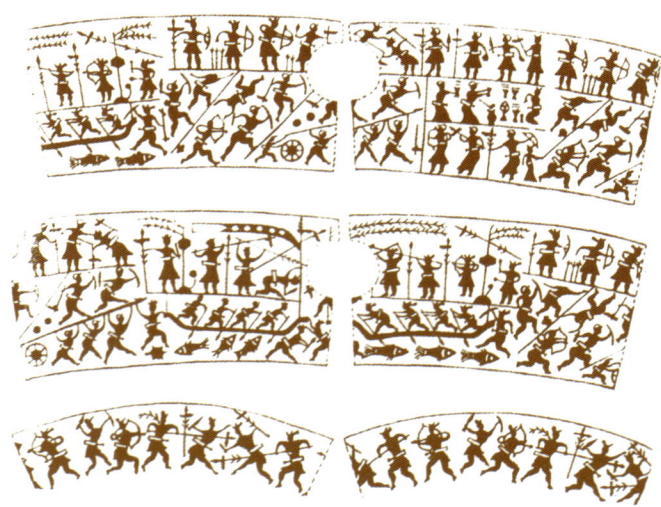

Decorative design on a bronze mirror from the Warring States Period (475–221 BC), depicting "martial beauty"

rope to tightly tie it around the animal's leg, thus tripping the animal. This ancient rope was the embryonic form of the wushu lasso weapons used by the later generations. Traditional wushu weapons such as "meteor hammer," "flying talon" and "flying hammer" all originated from it.

Due to development through primitive wars, the productive instruments that had been used for hunting gradually became refined into various weapons for fighting and killing people. Primitive military drills were gradually started in the form of "field hunting" and "armed dancing." "Field hunting" meant the training of soldiers to use various weapons and tactics, as well as to lead horses and chariots. "Armed dancing" referred to fighting between humans and wild animals, and between men and men, an imitation of hunting and battle scenes. The application of the experience of combat and killing in war to routine training was in essence the embryonic form of Chinese wushu.

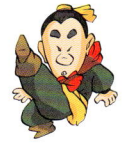

The rise of swordsmen and professional warriors

The making of swords through smelting has a history of over 3,000 years in China. The sword was a symbol of power as well as a protective weapon for rulers at the time of its first appearance. With improvements in smelting technique, the swords produced not only became more and more destructive to the human body, but also easier to carry, and thus came to be widely used in wars. About 2,200 years ago, ancient Chinese craftsmen could already make high-quality bronze swords. At the same time, swordsmen and professional warriors also arose among the people. In ancient China, when swordsmen and swordswomen were learning to use swords, they often encouraged themselves to study harder with the saying, "It takes 10 years to hone sword skills."

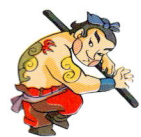

Heroine Hua Mulan

Women began to practice martial skills during a unique period through the years 220–589. Especially among matrilineal clan nationalities, women held high positions. When they came to the Central Plains for trade, they displayed their indomitable martial spirit. Some women of noble families mastered superb martial skills and even commanded troops to fight battles.

The inspiration for the leading role of Hua Mulan, in the Hollywood animated film *Mulan*, is from a famous real heroine from Chinese history. She lived during the Sui Dynasty (589–618). In those years, the tribes from the north often invaded the Central Plains, and the court sent troops to resist the invasions. Because her father was too old, Mulan stealthily disguised herself as a young man, so as to join the army on her father's behalf. She lived in the army for 12 years, and fought more than 100 battles, performing great meritorious service. Tales of her heroic deeds were passed down to later generations. For centuries, her reputation and deeds as a woman warrior were presented on stage. *Mulan Joins the Army* has been a popular classic opera or drama for generations.

Imperial examination specializing in military skills

Wu Zetian, the first empress in Chinese history, in 702 began to adopt a system of imperial examinations, specializing in military skills, as a way to select military personnel. This greatly promoted the popularization and improvement of the martial skills of military personnel and civilians. The examination consisted of three parts:

1. Military skills, mainly archery and spear skills;

2. Strength and endurance, namely weightlifting and load carrying;

3. Bodybuilding and conversation skills.

As it was more scientific and standardized than any previous method for selecting military personnel, her system continued to remain in use for more than 1,000 years, until it was abolished in 1905.

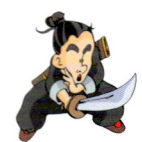

Chinese wushu and Japanese judo

Wushu routine techniques were greatly developed during the Song Dynasty (960–1279), mainly to meet demand for civilian entertainment as well as in military training. More attention began to be paid to bodywork, physical strength, rhythm and movement design. Each routine consisted of a starting position and a finishing position. Before a routine commenced, the practitioner had to make a fist-holding salutation as a sign of courtesy. This was an important symbol of maturity in the development of Chinese wushu.

Associations for practicing wushu were very popular among the common people in the Song Dynasty. The formation of associations created favorable conditions for the teaching, exchange and development of wushu among the people. Moreover, there were organized, regulated open wushu competitions with prizes, which had been rarely seen before. The thrilling description of how Yan Qing, a hero in *Outlaws of the Marsh*, dashed at his opponent using a stratagem on the stage, in the 74th chapter of the Chinese classic, is a vivid reflection of the popularity of wrestling in the Song Dynasty.

Japanese karate, judo and Chinese wushu are closely related in origins. The book *Quan Jing* (*Chinese Wushu Classic*), written by Ming Dynasty (1368–1644) grand general Qi Jiguang, was available in Japan around 1600. A Chinese martial expert of that time, Chen Yuanyun went in 1619 to Japan, where he taught Chinese wushu. Three of the students he taught created ancient Japanese jujitsu (later renamed 'judo') after learning Chinese martial arts. These three students were considered by later generations to be the founders of Japanese judo. Thus, Chen Yuanyun contributed to the founding of judo in Japanese history.

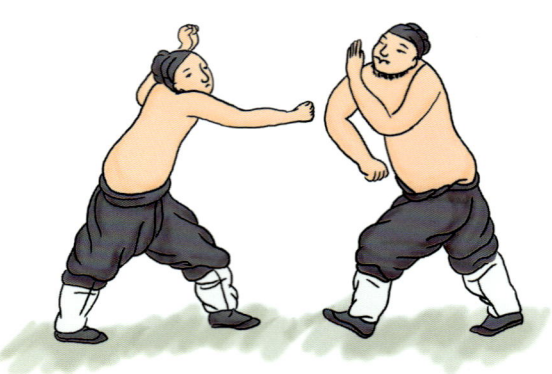

Thirty-two Changquan ("long boxing") technique from
Ming Dynasty General Qi Jiguang's *A Treatise on Efficiency*

Armed escorts—
real-life wushu masters

When we read a Chinese novel of chivalry or watch a kung fu film, we often come across agencies providing armed escorts and bodyguards. This phenomenon started in the late 17th century. Such agencies arose, grew and died out during the Qing Dynasty (1644–1911), through a history of more than 200 years, providing some fine pages in Chinese history. Such agencies not only provided economic security in the society, but also provided a form of livelihood to earn money through genuine skills for the wushu masters. Wushu gave the basic expertise on which the agency depended for its survival, and the armed escorts employed by the agency had to be wushu masters with special skills, otherwise they could not do the job. Among the different schools of wushu closely related with the armed escort agencies, Xingyi quan was the most influential school, and became most closely connected with the armed escort agencies. A Chinese wushu proverb says: "Taiji quan will not injure people after you practice it for 10 years, while Xingyi quan will kill people if you master it in one year." This shows the tremendous combat force of Xingyi quan.

"A man should seek self-improvement"

The Jingwu Sports Association was the largest and most influential wushu society in China. Its founder was the noted wushu master Huo Yuanjia. During the early years of the Republic of China (1911–1949), wushu masters emerged one after another, with Huo Yuanjia as an outstanding figure of this period. Because of his superb skills, he defeated or frightened off many Chinese and foreign challengers, and

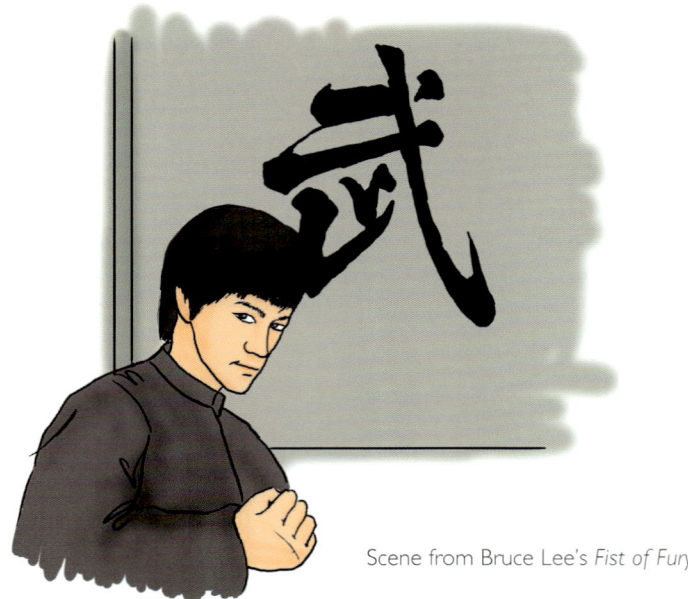

Scene from Bruce Lee's *Fist of Fury*

thus became a national hero. His heroic image is seen in many Chinese kung fu films. Bruce Lee, Jet Li and many other wushu masters have starred as Huo Yuanjia, portraying his superb skill in these films which depict the Chinese national spirit of striving for continual progress.

Bruce Lee

Bruce Lee devoted his legendary life to the international propagation of Chinese wushu, thus making a major contribution to its worldwide dissemination. Based on traditional Chinese wushu, Bruce Lee made an extensive study of boxing, karate, taekwondo, judo and Thai boxing, as well as French footwork techniques, and created his unique style of Jiequandao by assimilating their best points and discarding the bad points in a scientific way. At the time, he opened many Jiequandao clubs to teach wushu in the United States. Moreover, he also starred in the first Chinese kung fu film that was popular with cinemagoers worldwide. Many kung fu fans began to learn wushu precisely due to the influence of Bruce Lee's films.

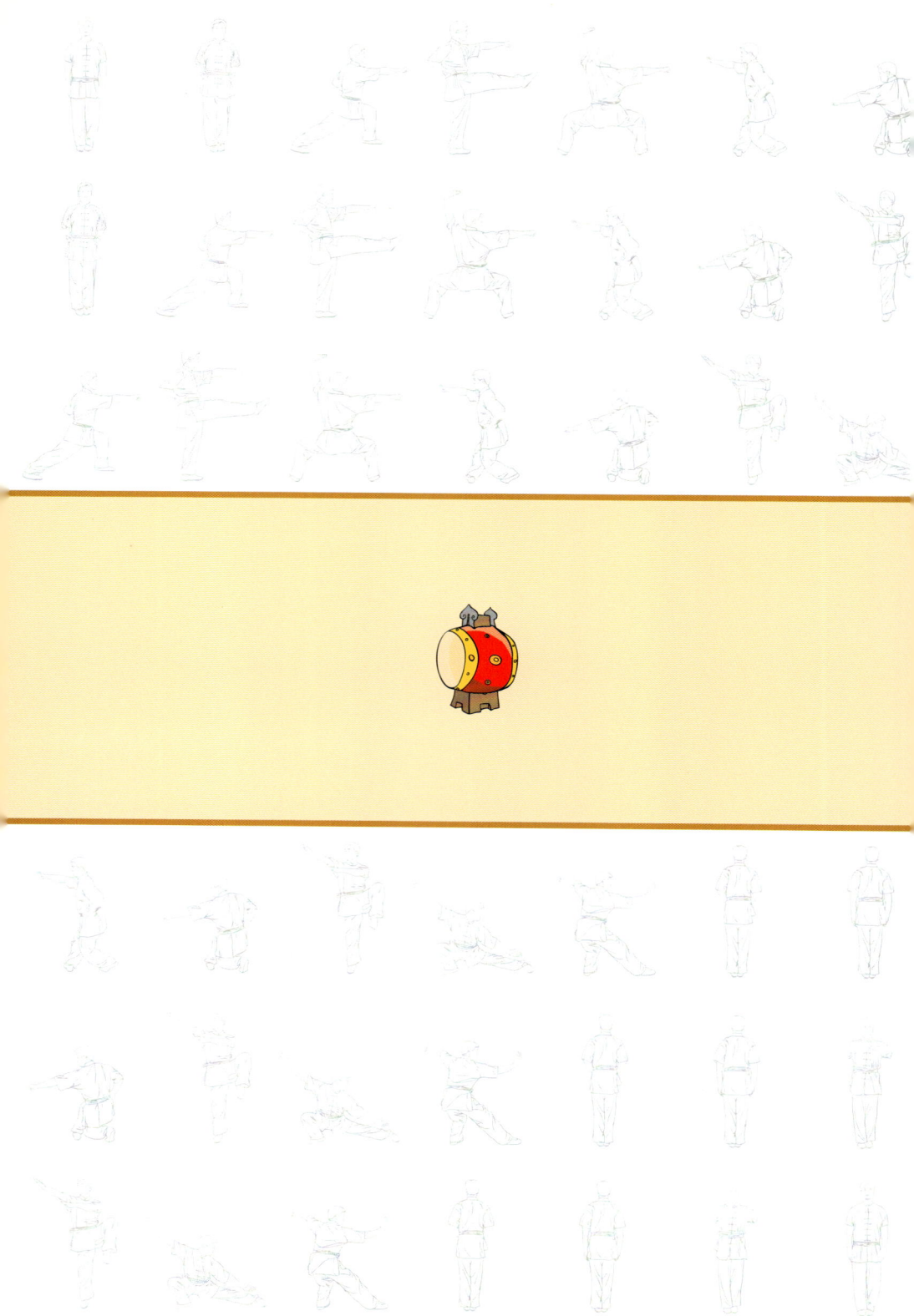

Key Words
to Open the Door to Wushu

Harmony between humans and nature

The fundamental concept in Chinese philosophy is of harmony between humans and nature. This is based on the belief that humans are an integral part of nature, and the supreme ideal of life being the conscious achievement of harmony between humans and nature.

The idea of "harmony between humans and nature" is reflected in wushu. It is demonstrated by the practitioners, who through wushu are in fact pursuing their own unity and harmony with nature. In concrete terms, wushu practitioners pay great attention to their harmony with the natural

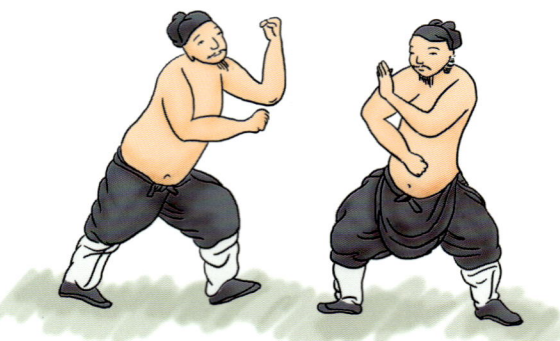

Thirty-two Changquan ("long boxing") technique from
Ming Dynasty General Qi Jiguang's *A Treatise on Efficiency*

environment, including the seasons, climate, geographical position and even direction, using different contents and methods suited to the time and location, and choosing quiet and beautiful places in which to practice.

For example, the practice of Xingyi quan must be matched with the different seasons to suit the rules of the seasons. In other words, when practicing it in spring, you should stress the release of inner energy (qi) and inner strength, and the movements should be slow and soft so that the main and collateral channels are gradually stretched. Summer is the time most suited for the release of strength, which will not strain or injure the muscles and bones. In autumn, the release of the strength should be less, with greater internal restraint. In winter when all things are desolate, inner strength should be hidden deeply and the practitioner should refrain from releasing it violently, so that it does not injure the muscles or lose vital energy.

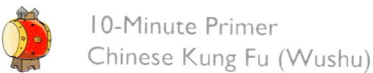
The concept of harmony between humans and nature emphasizes following nature as the model in the formulation process of wushu. For example, different forms of boxing were named after such animals, plants and astronomical phenomena as "tiger and crane," "eagle-claw," "monkey," "plum-blossom" "Big Dipper" and "evil star." The movements named after animals and plants include: "white crane spreading its wings," "black dragon emerging from water," "parting the wild horse's mane," "swallow touching the water," "roc spreading its wings," "ginger-twig boxing," "willow-leaf palm" and "plum-blossom stance," etc.

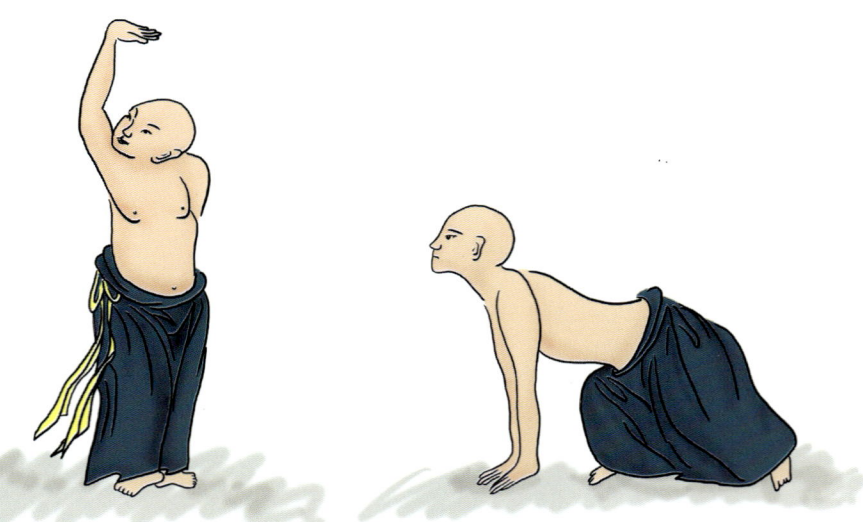

The stance of "plucking stars on each side" and the stance of "tiger springing on its prey" in Yi Jin Jing (Tendon-Muscle Strengthening Exercises)

Yin and Yang

Yin (lunar or negative) and Yang (solar or positive) constitute a very important part of traditional Chinese philosophy. For thousands of years, the concept of changes between Yin and Yang has exerted a profound influence on Chinese people's knowledge of the world and their daily life. It has also played a vitally important role in the theory and practice of wushu.

Yin and Yang in Wushu Theory

The Book of Changes says, "There is taiji in the changes, which is divided into two polarities." The two polarities are exactly Yin and Yang. The name of "Taiji quan" (shadow boxing, or Tai Chi Chuan) is precisely based on the theory that the taiji (the Supreme Ultimate) is divided into Yin and Yang, and Yin and Yang are integrated into the taiji. Wu Shu says in his book *Records of Arms*: "Attack is Yang, and defense is Yin." In *Theory of Taiji Quan*, Wang Zongyue wrote: "You should know about Yin and Yang: adhering means moving away, and moving away means adhering; Yin is not separated from Yang, and Yang is not separated from Yin. Only when Yin and Yang are put together, can you acquire the knowledge of strength." In *Illustrations of Chen-style Taiji quan*, Chen Xin said: "The key to Taiji quan lies in the two words: 'opening' and 'closing.' The wonderful thing about Yin and Yang as boxing lies in the way in which each is the root of the other."

Yin and Yang in wushu

In wushu drills, if the palm faces upward, it is called the "Yang hand"; and if the palm faces downward, it is called the "Yin hand." For example, when performing Yin *ba qiang* (Yin-handle spear), you often hold the spear with the palm facing downward, with the part of the hand between the thumb and the index finger backward, called "Yin hand."

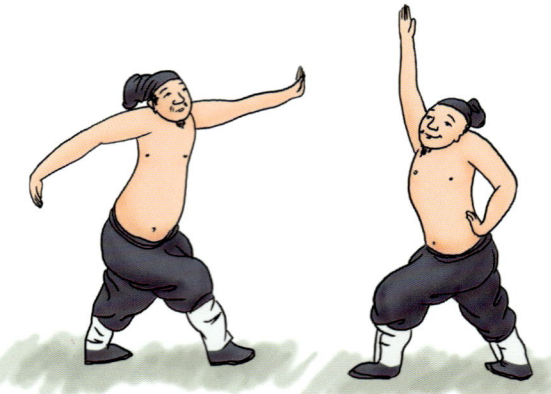

Thirty-two Changquan ("long boxing") technique from Ming Dynasty General Qi Jiguang's *A Treatise on Efficiency*

Explanations for the *Yin* and *Yang* Diagram of Taiji: a harmonious circular integrity is comprised of two *Yin* and *Yang* fish with corresponding heads and tails. The black fish has a white eye, and the white fish has a black eye. This implies that there is *Yang* in the *Yin*, and *Yin* in the *Yang*, and the *Yin* and *Yang* serve as each other's root. Between the two fish is an S-shaped curve. The curve in motion shows the beauty of spiraling changes on the one hand; and on the other, implies the dialectical idea of: "right first, if you want to move left; downward first, if you want to move upward; release first, if you want to withdraw; and close first, if you want to stretch open."

Theory of the five elements

The theory of the five elements has been prevalent since before the Qin Dynasty (221–206 BC). It became part of many aspects of the daily life of Chinese people. The theories of many types of quan or boxing in Chinese wushu involve the theory of the five elements. Five-element boxing in Xingyi quan is directly derived from the principle of each producing and being overcome by the other, in the theory of the five elements. Taiji quan also defines its five basic foot techniques as the five elements: "step in (fire), step back (water), step to the left (wood), step to the right (metal), and keep to the central position (earth)."

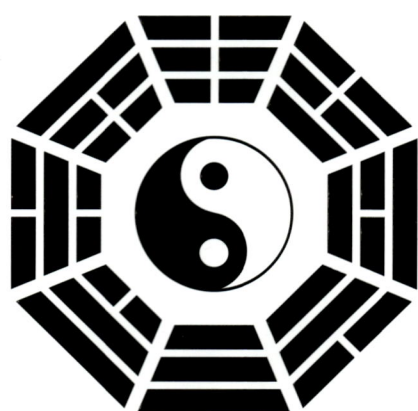

The development of wushu has a close bearing on Chinese medicine. The Yin and Yang theory of the five elements permeates all aspects of the theoretical system of Chinese medicine. The Yin and Yang theory of Chinese medicine deals with relations of opposition and restraint, serving as each other's root and using each other, growing and declining, while balancing and mutually transforming into each other between the functions of the human body and the natural foundation. The five elements theory of Chinese medicine exposes the functional structure of mutual growth and progressive mutual restraint between the major internal organs and tissues inside the human body, and between the major factors of the internal and external environments of the human body. The theory of Chinese medicine regards the heart, liver, spleen, lung and kidney as the five internal organs, drawing an analogy between them and the five elements, i.e. heart as fire, liver as wood, spleen as earth, lungs as metal, and kidneys as water. As the five elements each produce and are overcome by the others in a certain order, the five internal organs have the same relationships. Therefore, pathological changes in some internal organs in the human body often lead to the functional imbalance of other parts.

The relationships between five-element boxing and the five internal organs of the human body: "outward punch" improves the liver, "cannon hammer" improves the heart, "horizontal punch" improves the spleen, "straight arm chop" improves the lungs, and "drill chop" improves the kidneys.

Chen Wangting of the Ming Dynasty wrote in his book *Quan Jing* (*Boxing Classic*): "The five internal organs are the source and root of life. They are the heart, liver, spleen, lung and kidney. The heart belongs to fire, which gives rise to inflammation; the liver belongs to wood, which is either straight or bent in form; the spleen belongs to earth, which has a great momentum; the lung belongs to metal, which can be transformed into other things; the kidney belongs to water, which has the function of moistening other things..." "The functions of the five internal organs, solely motivated by the vital energy (*qi*), all cooperate with each other. All those who teach wushu cannot get away from this." We can thus see from this, the important place of the theory of the five elements in Taiji quan.

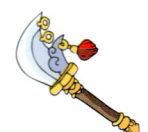

Wu de (martial virtues)

As an important military skill in ancient times, wushu required soldiers to be brave and stalwart. Though it is no longer prominent as a military skill today, martial arts are still considered to have great importance in the cultivation of fine moral character, through striving unceasingly to be stronger and enduring hardships. In wushu, both performers and spectators demonstrate their fearless spirit of going forward bravely. Even Taiji quan, which is performed gently and slowly, also stresses the spirit of vigor and promise.

On the relationship between hard work and success, Bruce Lee said: "If you want to be above ordinary people, you must be ready at all times to take arduous and tedious training as your greatest pleasure. The more ready you are to accept such torment, the more possible it is to become a success." The process of working diligently is in fact a process of self-emancipation. Through the tempering of the body and the mind, you will gradually release yourself from the yoke of techniques in terms of your body and from the shackles of knowledge in terms of your mind, so that there will exist no more obstacles between the body and the mind, and the body and the mind become integrated as one. Superb skill enables the body to freely convey your innermost thoughts. In fact, through persistent tempering, you should learn to express yourself completely and fully.

The two characters 武德 (*wu de*) mean "martial virtues."
"Learn virtues first, before learning wushu."
"Stop fighting" is the meaning of *wu*, while "respect martial virtue" is the meaning of *de*.

Gongfu salutation

The traditional gongfu salutation features a tight right fist, which signifies the respect given to martial arts, a flat left hand with bent thumb, which implies modesty to accept instruction and avoid conceit, while the other four fingers of the left hand, held closely together, represent the solidarity and progress of the martial arts community. The left hand should cover the right fist, which represents honoring martial virtues, making friends on the stage of martial arts, and not allowing the strong to bully the weak. The bent arms form a circle, which implies harmony and solidarity among the martial arts community.

"Learn the salutation before learning the art."

Martial virtues:
- Keep your promises
- Be strict with yourself in observing laws and discipline
- Take pleasure in helping others
- Respect the teacher and cherish the students; always be courteous
- Be humble and sincere
- Be amiable and accessible
- Be modest and careful
- Show a strong will both in severe winter cold and intense summer heat
- Continue to improve
- Demonstrate filial piety, fraternity and justice
- Help those in distress and in poverty

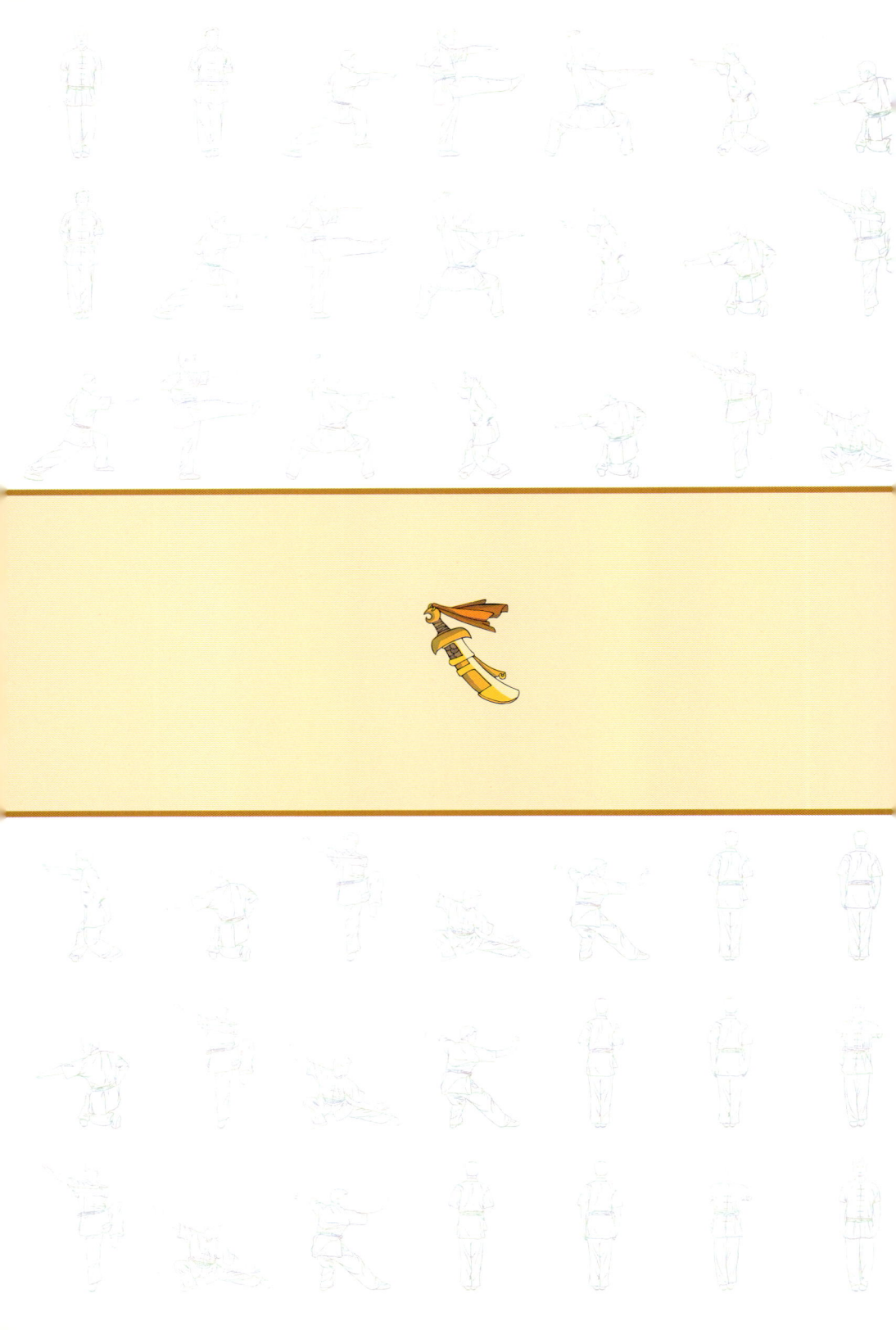

The Family Tree of Wushu

Chinese wushu has a long and flourishing history, rich in content.

Schools of wushu

The schools of wushu refer to the different sects of wushu, which were formed according to the various distinctive characteristics of their techniques and styles. There are many versions of classification of the schools of wushu. Here we will just touch on classification according to the family names of the founders of the schools.

Chinese people attach great importance to ties of blood, families and kinship. Wushu has been handed down and developed with families as the basic units. Hitherto, some clans still control the nuclear skills of their boxing schools, and have kept them secret.

The traditional Chinese method of passing on wushu skills is face-to-face exhortation between the master and the apprentice, and strict one-to-one individual teaching. The traditional forms of address are: "teacher-father" (a man as affectionate and dignified as a father), and "pupil" or "disciple" (as filial and submissive as a child).

The implications of 门 *men* (society), 派 *pai* (school or sect), 家 *jia* (family) and 式 *shi* (style) in Chinese wushu

门 *men* (society) in Chinese wushu refers to a wushu society or club, or an association, formed by a set of people who believe in or venerate a type of gongfu and meet to learn it together. For example, the wushu group that specializes in the Shaolin quan is called the "Shaolin Society," while the group specializing in Bagua zhang (Eight-trigram Palm) is known as the "Bagua Society."

派 *pai* (school or sect) in Chinese wushu refers to a wushu school in which some wushu masters made innovations and developments on the basis of the original routines practiced, and after repeated study and practice or even generations of practice, formulated a wushu system with a unique style that was different from others in the same or other societies, but without any changes in its original foundation. For example, Shaolin quan is divided into different schools of Henan, Fujian, Guangdong, Emei and Wudang; and Taiji quan is divided into the five schools of Chen, Yang, Sun, Wú and Wǔ styles.

家 *jia* (family) can be exemplified by the Hong, Yu and Kong families or clans of Henan's Shaolin school, whose study and practice of Shaolin quan have reached a very high level, and who have been very influential and innovative in carrying out the Shaolin school tradition.

式 *shi* (style) has two meanings: first, referring to separate wushu movements; second, the unique style of wushu movement, differing in form from that practiced in the same school yet with the same essentials, as developed by extremely expert and innovative wushu masters—the Chen style, Yang style, Sun style, Wú Yu Xiang style and Wǔ styles of Taiji quan.

Classification of wushu by content

Chinese wushu can be divided into routine forms and combat forms, as well as various specialized forms of exercises related to the two.

Routine forms

The routines are a unique form of exercise in Chinese wushu. Wushu routines refer to a form of sport in which a number of movements are arranged in a given sequence for exercise.

Wushu routines can be divided into three types: solo, dual and group exercises.

Solo exercises include (1) bare-handed boxing and (2) use of weapons.

(1) "Chinese boxing" refers to solo bare-handed exercises in the form of a routine.

Changquan or "long boxing" is the most popular and orthodox school among the northern wushu schools. It is characterized by limber postures, and flexible, quick, rhythmical and forceful movements, which include leaps, jumps, and tumbling, as well as somersaults.

Xiangxing quan or "imitation boxing" is a type of boxing that imitates the skills, specialties and forms of a particular animal or imitates the forms of movements of a particular person, combined with attack and defense techniques. "Imitation boxing" is characterized by imitating the form as the posture and the use of the form to express ideas, appearing vivid and lifelike.

Stage photo of Jackie
Chan's "drunkard's boxing"

The major popular styles are: mantis boxing, monkey boxing, eagle-claw boxing, snake boxing, drunkard's boxing, etc. Mantis-style boxing is the most representative of all "imitation boxing" styles. The mantis has two long and big forelegs resembling two big axes. The front section of its foreleg has a hook, and the middle section is large

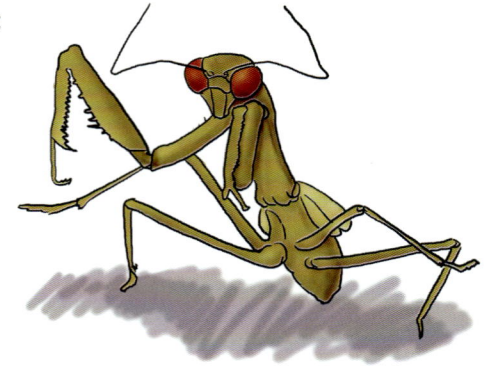

"Mantis boxing"

with many hooked thorns. It twists its waist and turns its head with the rear legs touching the ground. Its movements are very agile. It is brave when it captures other insects for food or guards against enemy attack. "Mantis-style boxing" imitates the movements, manners and combat techniques of a mantis, combined with the attack and defense techniques of wushu. It is an offensive form of boxing, and has enjoyed a long-standing reputation for its quick, powerful, graceful and varied movements.

Apart from "imitation boxing," there are many other boxing styles and movements that are derived from the movements of animals. For example, the traditional routine of "12 Forms," which constitutes a very important part of

Xingyi quan, imitates the forms of 12 different animals and their fighting techniques. A few movements of Taiji quan were also named after animal imagery, such as "white crane spreading its wings," "step back and repulse the monkey," "white snake spitting out its tongue," and "part the wild horse's mane."

(2) "Weapons" refers to forms of exercise using wushu weapons. They are divided into: short weapons, including broadsword, sword, and dagger; long weapons, or spear and cudgel; double weapons, as in double broadswords, double swords and double hooks; and soft weapons, such as the nine-section whip and rope dart.

Moreover, there is an unusual weapon form in Chinese wushu—hidden weapons.

"Hidden weapons" refer to a type of weapon that is hidden before it is thrown or shot. It has the feature of attacking an unprepared opponent.

Combat forms

Combat event refers to combat forms between two people conducted according to prescribed rules under certain conditions. It includes free sparring, pushing hands and short weapons.

Exercises

Exercises are very important in Chinese wushu. There is a popular saying: "If you do not do exercises in practicing wushu, you will achieve nothing when you grow old." All hitting or striking movements, such as hand striking, foot kicking, shoulder bumping, buttock pushing, head butting, broadsword chopping, spear piercing, sword pointing or cudgel sweeping, must develop considerable power to strike and resist striking without exception. The only way for wushu practitioners to achieve such ability is by doing the exercises. You must endure the hardship of doing the exercises, and persist in doing them for years without interruption. Therefore, the exercises not only help to improve performance and combat skills, but will also help to steel your indomitable will.

The exercises in Chinese wushu mainly comprise exercises of internal power and exercises of external power, i.e., internally, the spirit, vital energy and mind; externally, the muscles, bone and skin.

Chinese wushu practitioners in ancient times believed that there are three treasures in Heaven: the sun, the moon and the stars; three treasures on the Earth: water, fire and wind; and three treasures in the human body: spirit, vital energy and mind.

Some of the exercises in wushu have developed or evolved into forms of mass sports, such as the "dragon dance," "lion dance," "shuttlecock kicking" and "rope skipping."

"Lion dance" was an ancient folk pastime in China. It was first started for driving away evils and ghosts. Lion dancers often have good wushu skills and techniques. "Lion dances" are very popular in overseas Chinese communities. In performing the lion dance, dancers in northern China mainly perform separate or small set of movements, while those in southern China mostly perform fairly complicated sets. The southern dancers often try to catch green cabbages, the name for which sounds like "fortune" in Chinese, and the northern dancers perform dancing skills and play with colorful silk balls. There are more than 100 different kinds of lion dance performances in China.

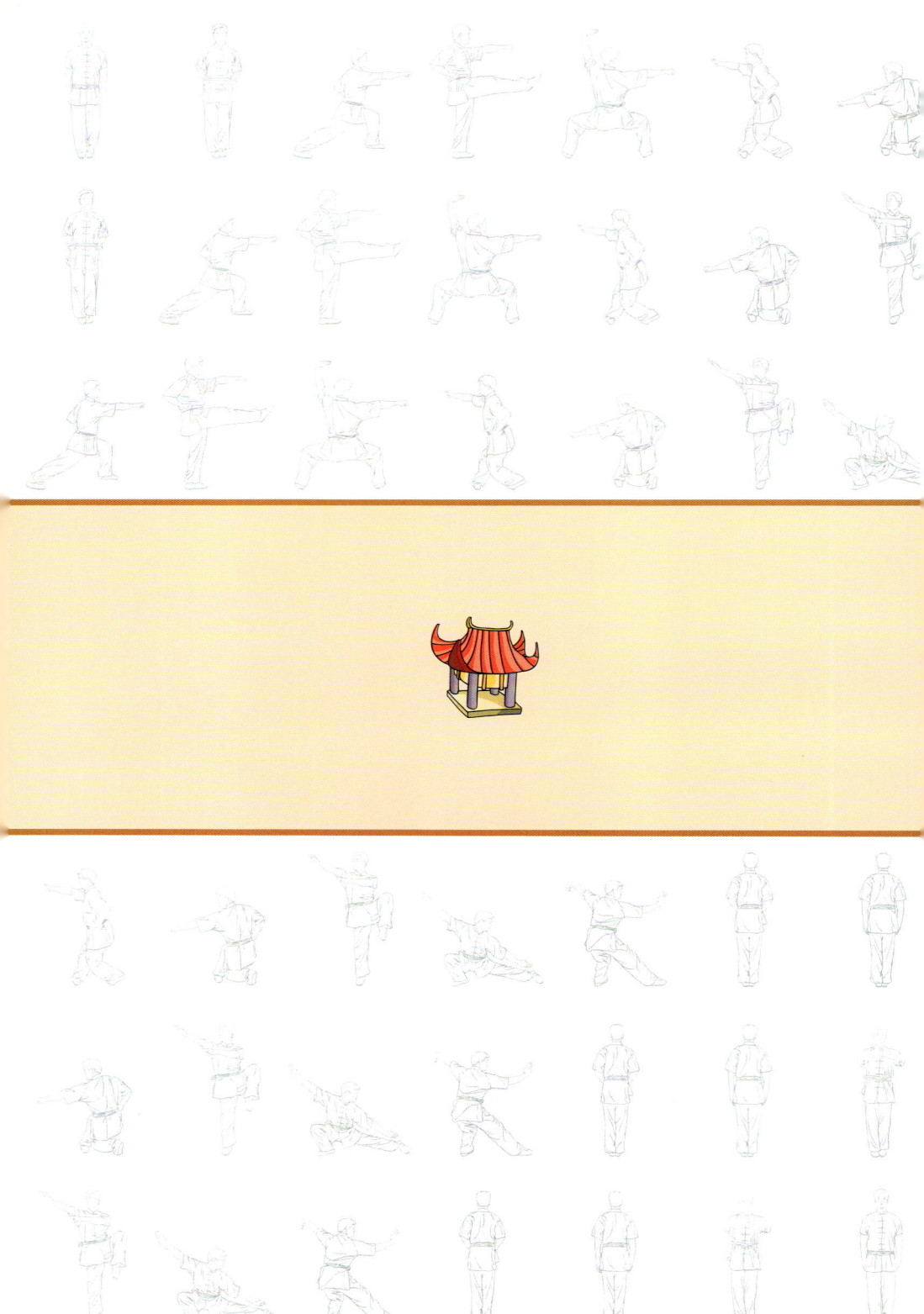

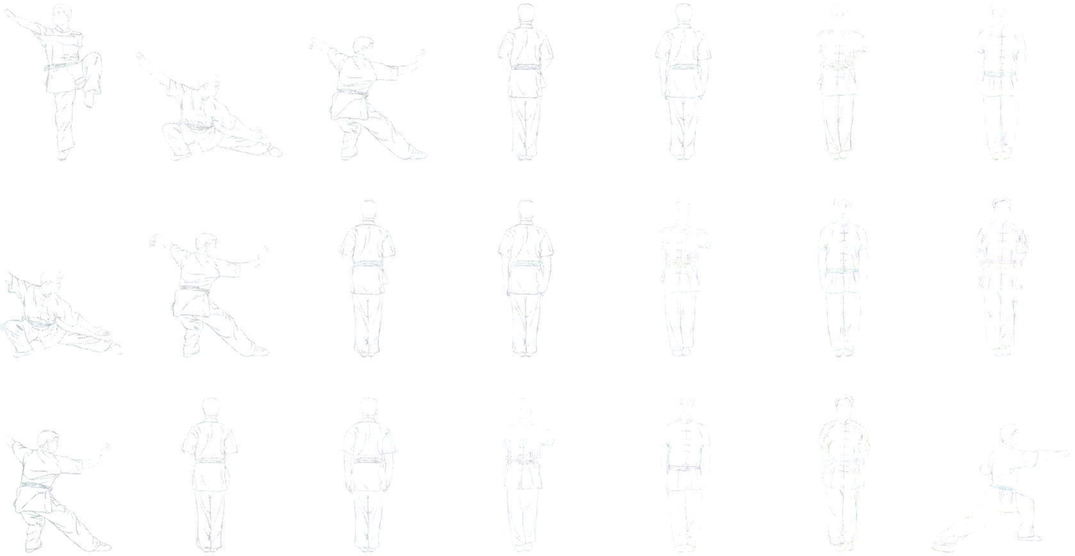

Chinese Wushu and Health

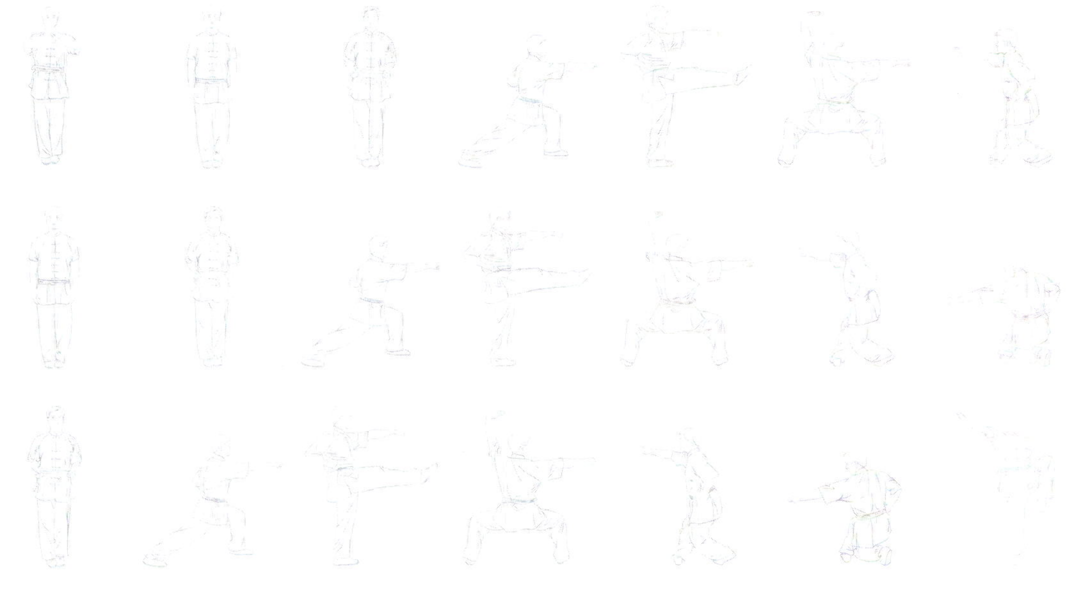

Wushu health effects

Wushu can help:

- Maintain and develop the normal posture of the body;
- Strengthen the muscles and bones;
- Improve the function of the respiratory system;
- Make blood circulation smoother;
- Improve digestion;
- Improve the endocrine system;
- Improve metabolism;
- Make sense organs keener and movements more harmonious;
- Improve immunity functions;
- Inspire wisdom and improve thinking.

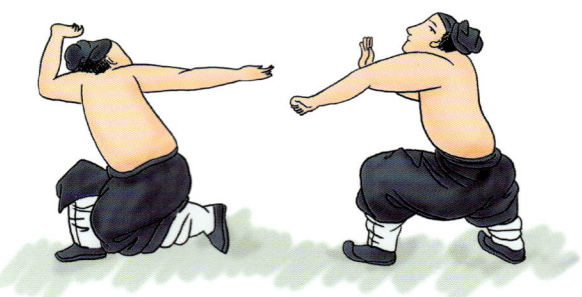

Thirty-two Changquan ("long boxing") technique from
Ming Dynasty General Qi Jiguang's *A Treatise on Efficiency*

"Hitting the vital points" in wushu

Traditional Chinese medicine believes that there are passages in the human body through which vital energy (*qi*) circulates to regulate bodily functions and the collaterals that branch out from the main passages. Along the main and collateral passages are distributed the meeting points of the passages of blood and *qi*, which are known as the "vital points" or "acupuncture points." When these special points are hit suddenly from outside, the passages are blocked or severed, thus hindering the normal circulation of the blood and *qi*, and affecting the normal physiological functions of the vital energy, blood and internal organs. The harmful physiological reactions produced after striking the vital points are mainly: dizziness, unconsciousness or numbness. Sometimes, even life is endangered when these key "points" are hit.

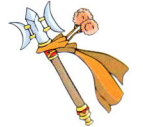

Wushu and psychological health

Concentration power

A wushu routine often consists of a dozen or even several dozen movements. This requires the practitioners to concentrate their attention and coordinate the changing movements, breathing and rhythms, without any distracting thoughts.

The exercises for internal power in wushu, such as Yi Jin Jing of Shaolin quan and *qigong*, have unique curative effects, helping to ease the tensions of modern people, alleviate mental stress, and treat neuroses, depression, weakness, world-weariness, or other sub health problems.

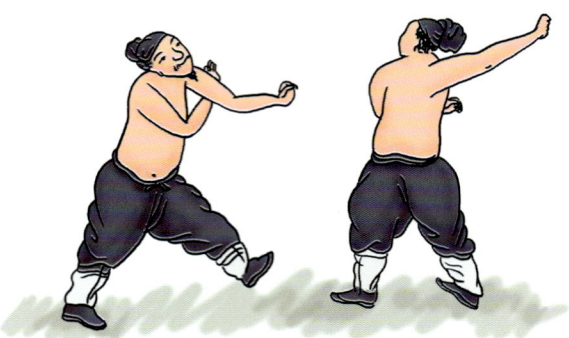

Thirty-two Changquan ("long boxing") technique from
Ming Dynasty General Qi Jiguang's *A Treatise on Efficiency*

Ability to maintain calm

Because wushu practitioners must keep calm and use stillness to control movement when they do exercises, they will gradually cultivate an attitude of serenity. When they relate with others and conduct themselves in society, they begin also to acquire the habit of solving problems in objective and rational ways, guided objectively in observing things and not influenced by self-image.

Increased self-confidence

People who do not have self-confidence think that they are below or inferior to others, and therefore easily become disappointed, timid and afraid, often trying to avoid problems that arise. Some people think that because they are not in good health they will never achieve anything, and thus become dejected and weak, or even acquire bad habits. Wushu can not only keep people in good health, but also help them to defend themselves. Long-time practice not only enables them to increase self-confidence and overcome any sense of inferiority, but also improve their ability to make correct judgments, tell right from wrong and tolerate hardship and pain, thus improving their psychological health.

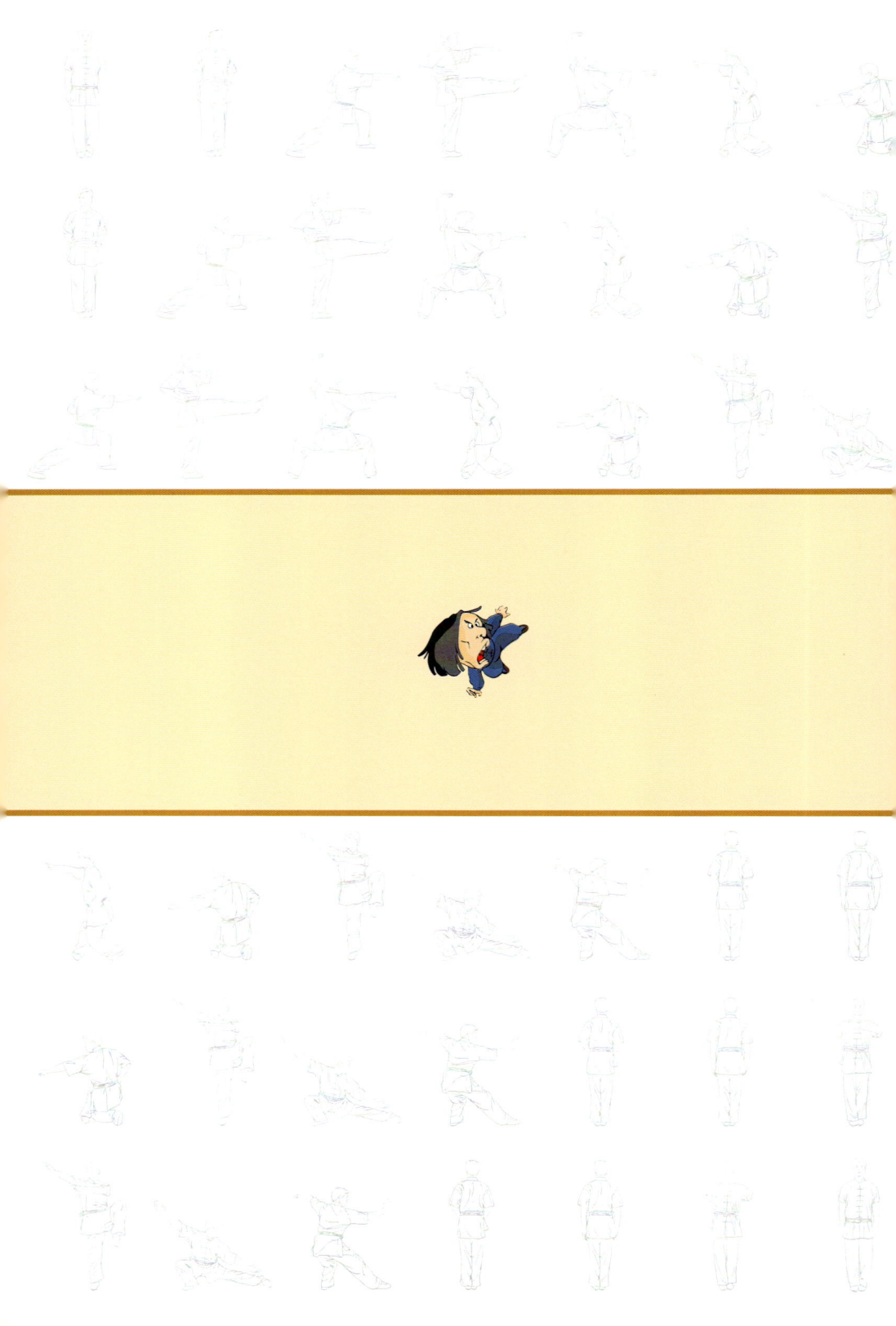

Beginning to Become Bruce Lee

Five-stance quan is a routine composition of the five most important and distinctive stances in wushu, combined with leg techniques, fist techniques and palm techniques. It is short, terse, compact and cohesive. It is an important part of the fundamental exercises of wushu.

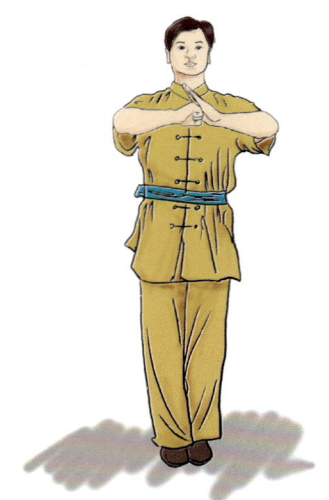

The five stances

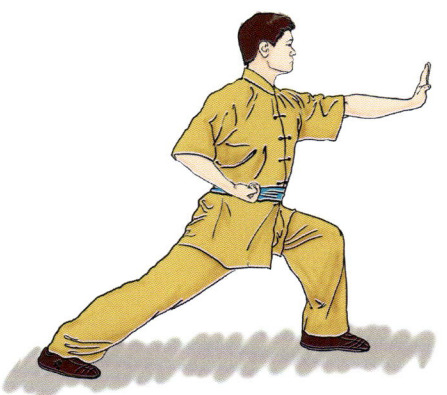

Bow stance

Movements: Keep the front foot slightly pointed inward, the entire sole on the ground, in half squat with the knee bent, the thigh parallel to the ground, the knee perpendicular to the instep; keep the rear leg straight, toes inward, the entire sole on the ground, and the upper body facing forward.

Key points: Chest forward, back straight, front leg bent, and rear leg straightened.

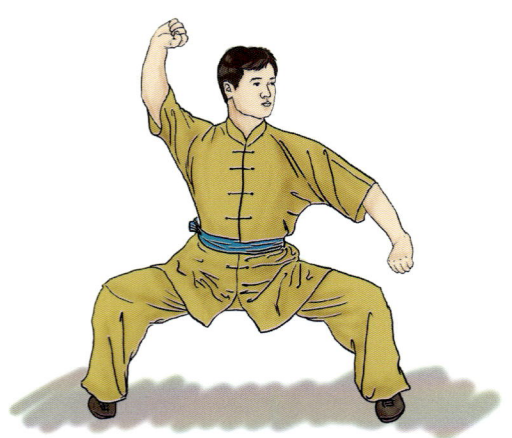

Horse stance

Movements: Keep the feet apart, with the distance between them about three and a half times the length of the foot, toes pointing forward, in a half squat with knees bent, thighs parallel to the ground, eyes to the left, holding the fists as in the picture.

Key points: Head erect, chest forward, back straight, and feet pointing forward.

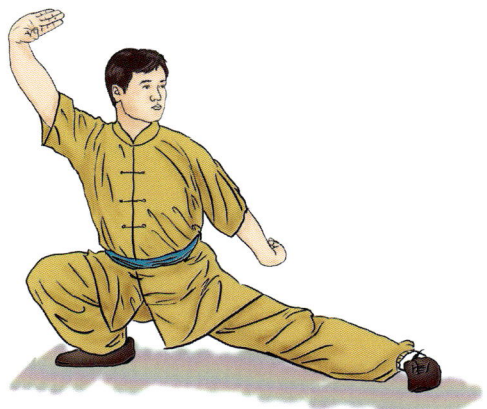

Crouch stance

Movements: Keep one leg in a squatting position, thigh and shin against each other, the entire sole on the ground, knee and toes pointing slightly outward; the other leg stretched out, close to the ground, the entire foot on the ground, and toes pointed inward.

Key points: Chest forward, back straight, hips wide, and the entire sole on the ground.

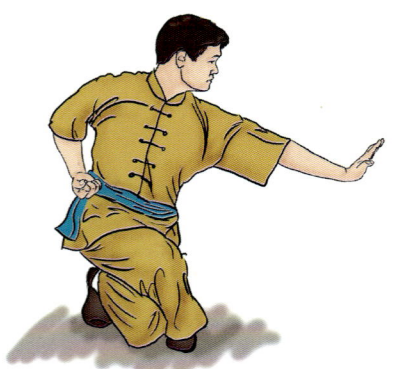

Cross-legged sitting stance

Movements: Keep the legs bent and crossed in a squatting position, the sole of the forward foot on the ground, toes outward, the heel of the rear foot off the ground, and the outer sides of the buttocks closely against the back shins.

Key points: Chest forward, back straight, and both legs closely against each other.

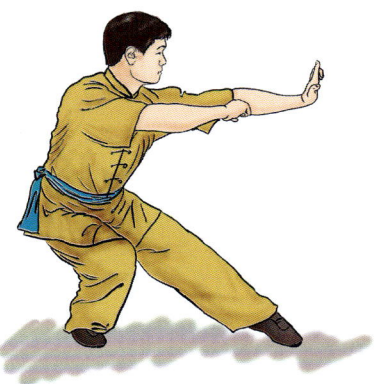

Empty stance

Movements: Keep the rear foot obliquely forward, knee bent in a half squat and the entire sole on the ground and toes pointing outward; keep the forward leg slightly bent, instep straightened, and toes lightly touching the ground.

Key points: Chest forward, back straight, body weight on the rear leg, and forward leg unsupported.

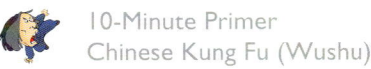
Fist

Movements: Clench the five fingers, thumb covering the second phalanges of the index finger and the middle finger.

Key points: Clench the fist tightly, with the front of the fist flat and wrist straight.

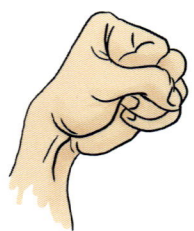

Palm

Movements: Keep the four fingers straight and together, with the thumb bent closely against the palm side of the hand.

Key points: Keep the palm fully open, with the fingers stretched.

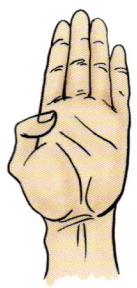

Hook

Movements: Keep the fingers together into a hook, with the wrist bent.

Key points: Bend the wrist.

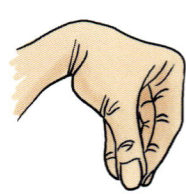

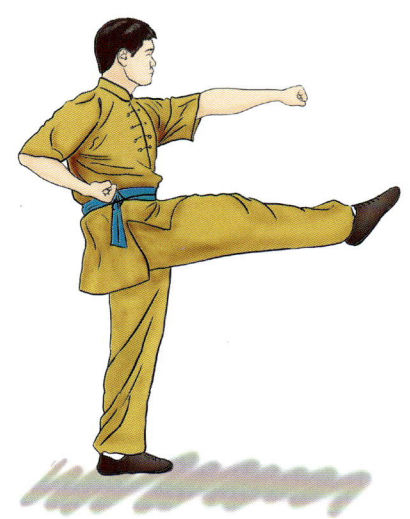

Snap kick

Movements: Keep the supporting leg straight or slightly bent, while the other leg moves from being bent to kicking forward, with the instep flat and the power reaching the toes.

Key points: Draw the buttocks back, and kick with explosive force.

The names and order of the movements of the five-stance quan

- Starting position
- Punching fist, in a bow stance
- Punching fist, with a snap kick
- Blocking palm, in a horse stance
- Pressing and punching fist, in a cross-legged sitting stance
- Piercing palm, with knee raised in a crouch stance
- Snapping palm, in an empty stance
- Keep feet together, with fists held on hips
- Closing form

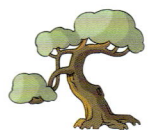

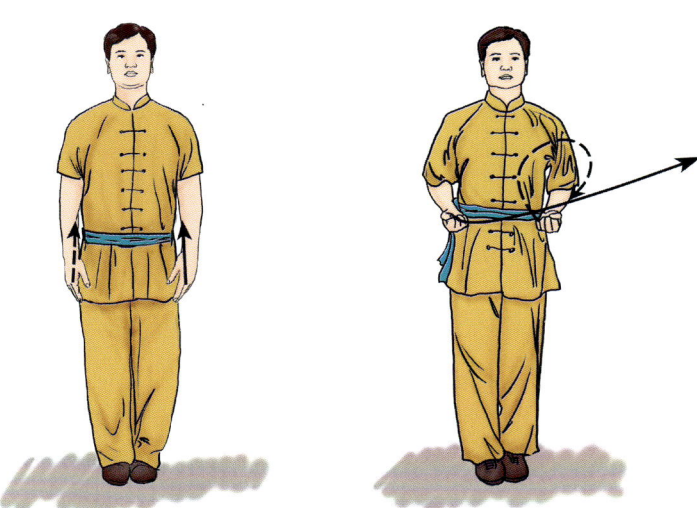

Starting position

Stand erect, with both hands down by your sides. Keep the feet together, with fists held on hips.

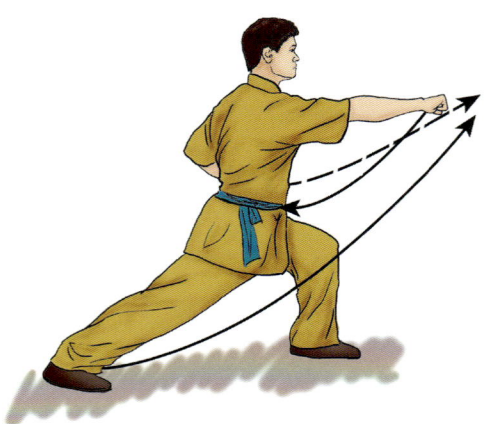

Punching fist, in a bow stance

Step forward with the left foot to form a left bow stance. Brush to the left with the left hand, draw it back to the waist, and hold the fist; punch with the right fist. Eyes in front.

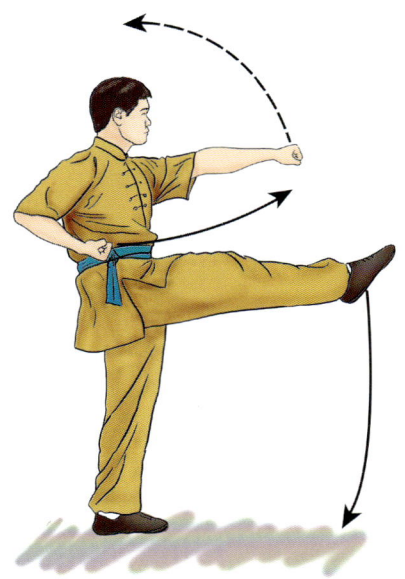

Punching fist, with a snap kick

Shifting your weight forward, kick forward with the right leg and a snap. At the same time, punch with the left fist while pulling the right fist back. Eyes in front.

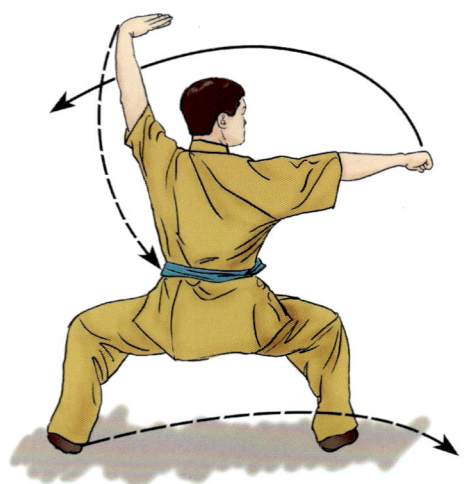

Blocking palm, in a horse stance

The right foot firmly on the ground, turn the body to the left 90 degrees, and then squat down to a horse stance. At the same time, open the left fist into a palm, block upward with arm bent, and punch with the right fist. Eyes to the right.

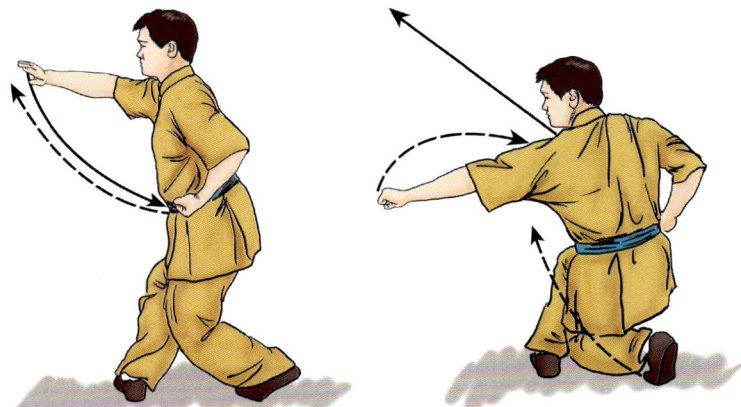

Pressing and punching fist, in a cross-legged sitting stance

Move the left foot backward to cross behind the right foot. At the same time, open the right fist into a palm, and press it downward to the left, with the outer side of the palm forward, turn the body to the left 90 degrees, and draw the left fist back, with eyes on the right fist. While continuing the above movement, bend both legs into a cross-legged sitting stance, punch with the left fist and draw the right fist back, eyes on the left fist.

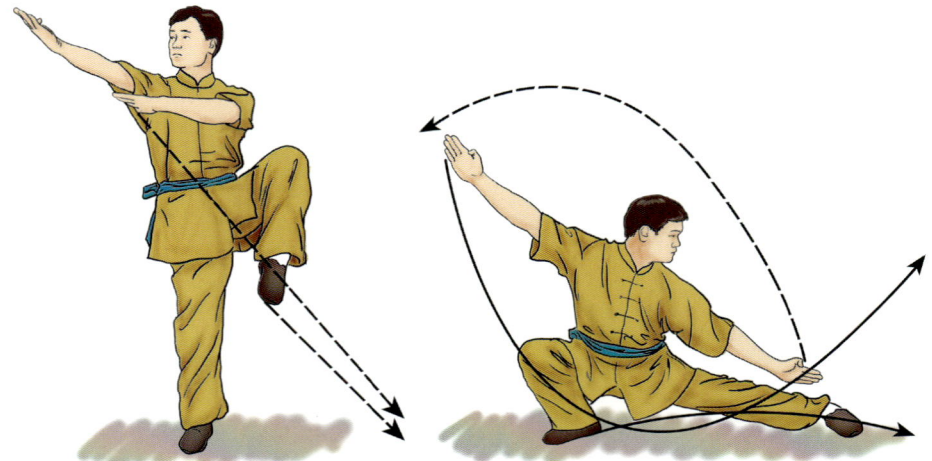

Piercing palm, with knee raised in a crouch stance

Rise on both legs, and turn the body to the left. Immediately open the left fist into a palm and draw it back to under the right armpit. Open the right fist into a palm, and slide it above the back of the left hand, palm upward. At the same time, raise the left leg with knee bent, eyes on the right hand. While continuing the above movement, firmly place the left foot on the ground to form a crouch stance. Keep the fingers of the left palm facing the front, and pierce the palm along the inner side of the left leg to the left instep, eyes on the left palm.

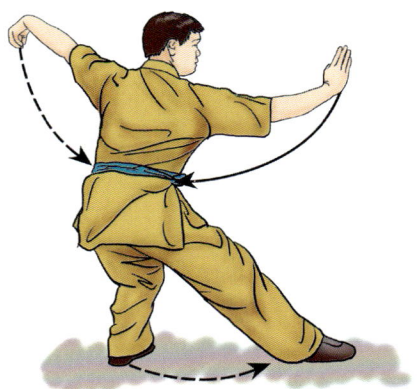

Snapping palm, in an empty stance

Bend the left leg forward in a bow stance, and move the right foot forward to form an empty right stance. At the same time, move the left hand backward in an arc to form a hooked hand, and move the right hand along the outer side of the right leg in an upward snapping palm, with eyes in front.

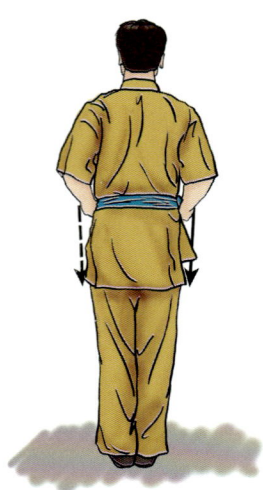

Keep feet together, with fists held on hips

Move the left foot towards the right foot, to keep them together. At the same time, maintain the left hooked hand and change the right palm into a fist. Pull them back and hold them on the hips, with eyes in front.

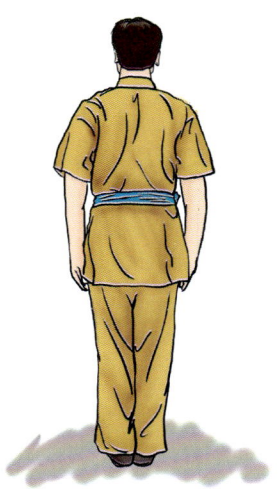

Closing form

Open both fists into palms, and place them back down by the sides of the body.